PERSONAL YOGA PRACTICE
JOURNAL

Introduction by Olga Kabel, RYT, C-IAYT

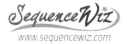

www.sequencewiz.com

WHY PRACTICE YOGA AT HOME?

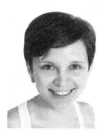 Hi there! My name is Olga Kabel; I am a yoga teacher and yoga therapist. I have been practicing yoga since 2000 and teaching since 2001, so it's been a while. In all those years my personal yoga practice had carried me through both mundane and challenging times. Over the years my practice has evolved, expanded and contracted based on the issues I was dealing with, but I always knew that I could come back to it any time to move, breathe and reassess.

The *Personal Yoga Practice Journal* is my effort to support you in developing or reigniting your home yoga practice, so that you, too, have a place to go whenever you need to reconnect to your body, get a clearer picture of what's going on in your life, and correct course when necessary.

As you know, consistency is key when it comes to practicing yoga. According to Patanjali's Yoga Sutras, "The speed of your progress on the path of change is in direct proportion to your faith and the effort you put into it" (Sutra 1-22). If you are only mildly interested in transformation and attend to it occasionally, it will take you a lo-o-ong time to get there. If your interest is strong and your practice consistent, then you will progress faster. And, of course, if you are completely committed to your goal and practice your yoga on and off the mat all the time, the transformation will be rapid.

My teacher Gary Kraftsow often compares regular home yoga practice to flossing. He jokes that you should only floss around the teeth that you want to keep. You floss to both get rid of the waste (food particles) and to keep your teeth and gums healthy. Similarly, regular home practice helps you let go of things you don't need (tension, sluggishness, restlessness, etc.) and keeps you healthy and more content.

What is it about regular home practice that makes it so important? If you are a yoga student, how do you want to feel when you start your day? I have yet to meet a student who PREFERS to feel grumpy, stiff and restless in the morning. You would probably want to start your day feeling comfortable in your body, energized and focused. Even a very simple yoga practice can do that for you.

What if you are dealing with a specific issue, like tension, a health problem, an undesirable pattern of behavior? Then an appropriate regular yoga practice becomes even more important. Remember Einstein's definition of insanity? It's "doing the same thing over and over again and expecting different results." If your previous patterns of movement or behavior got you in trouble, how are you going to replace them with a more desirable pattern if you don't practice?

If you are a yoga teacher, regular home practice becomes more of a necessity. As yoga teachers, we are not only responsible for our own sense of wellbeing, but also for the kind of energy and attitude we bring to our students. Your home yoga practice is an opportunity to, among other things:

- Take care of yourself - physically, energetically and mentally;
- To experiment with tools and techniques that you might eventually teach to your students;
- To inspire you, keeping your teaching fresh, potent and versatile;
- To help you connect to your students;
- To remind you why you are doing this in the first place.

Home yoga practice is not just about "limbering up" for the day ahead, but about setting the tone for the entire day. And your practice doesn't have to be perfect; in fact, it doesn't have to be anything. As long as it's mindful, it matters. We all have different ideas about what our home yoga practice SHOULD look like, and often those ideas can become a hindrance. If you believe that your practice should be at least one hour long, you will be less likely to do it, since it's not easy to carve out an hour every single day. There is a saying: "Doing nothing changes nothing, doing something changes everything," which is very true when it comes to a home yoga practice. If you resolve to do something (no matter how small) every day, you are more likely to continue and turn it into a healthy habit.

The *Personal Yoga Practice Journal* will help you build your yoga practice into your day and keep track of your progress. You can plan the direction of your yoga practice for the next month using the 30 DAYS OF YOGA planning pages. It is useful if you are trying to investigate a specific set of practices, test certain techniques or consistently work on a chronic problem. Otherwise you can record your practices day-to-day, attending to the needs that arise.

When you decide on what kind of yoga practices to choose, there are three things to consider:

1. You are a multidimensional human being, which means that your wellbeing is linked to several layers of your system, not just the physical body, and your yoga practice needs to reflect that. **The Panchamaya model** is an excellent yogic guide that describes five main layers of the human system, what it takes to have balance on each one of those levels, and which tools are most effective for achieving that balance.
2. Your needs depend on your stage of life. Are you in a sunrise, midday or sunset stage? The viniyoga **Age model** describes each life stage and yoga practices that are the most relevant to each stage.
3. Every yoga practice needs to be purposeful. There are **Ten types of practices** based on the things that you want to accomplish. Choosing the right one will help you get the best results.

Your yoga practice is not something separate from your daily life; it can become its integral part. It can become the support structure that gives you physical stability, consistent energy and a focused mind to enable you to do whatever it is you want to do with your life. It can also become a safety net that will catch you when life gets rough. There is no better time to begin than now.

THE PANCHAMAYA MODEL

Modern science has been slow to recognize the intimate connection between our physical structure, physiology, mind, emotions and spiritual longings; when health problems arise they are usually treated on one level only. The yoga tradition, on the other hand, recognizes that our systems are multidimensional and interconnected. Therefore, if we are planning to be vibrant, healthy human beings, we need to consider all the components that make up our systems: physical structure, physiological processes, the content of our minds, our ideas and attitudes toward our surroundings and our sense of connection to other people, society and the Universe.

The Panchamaya model (also called the **Five Koshas**) is a way to organize our thinking when it comes to different layers of our systems. Everything you've ever learned about yoga fits somewhere within the Panchamaya model; it is a yogic view of how things work within our bodies and minds. This model is extremely useful (and even necessary) when we are trying to understand what's happening within ourselves or our students. True knowledge does not lie in mastering difficult postures or complicated techniques. It lies in developing an insightful and intimate knowledge of how our systems function and learning the tools to fine tune them when necessary.

Here is how those five dimensions (or 5 bodies) are described in a yoga classic, *The Taittiriya Upanishad*:

> "Human beings consist of a **material body** build from the food they eat. Those who care for this body are nourished by the universe itself"
>
> "Inside there is another **body made of life energy**. It fills the physical body and takes its shape. Those who treat this vital force as divine, experience excellent health and longevity because this energy is the source of physical life."
>
> "Within the vital force is yet another **body**, this one **made of thought energy**. Those who understand and control the mental body are no longer afflicted by fear."
>
> "Deeper still lies another **body comprised of intellect**. Those who establish their awareness here free themselves from unhealthy thoughts and actions, and develop the self-control necessary to achieve their goals."
>
> "Hidden inside is yet a subtler **body, composed of pure joy**. It is experienced as happiness, delight and bliss."

Yoga is a unique discipline that has developed specific tools for addressing imbalances in each one of these dimensions. You don't take Pepto Bismol to treat a headache – in the same way the selection of yogic tools needs to be appropriate for the issue that you are dealing with. Our job as yoga teachers is to continuously refine our skills and our understanding of each one of those five dimensions and apply our knowledge in a way that is appropriate for the student.

THE PANCHAMAYA MODEL

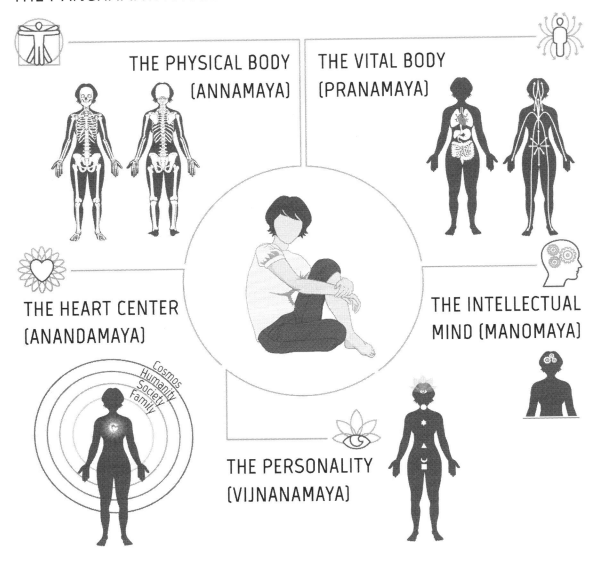

THE PHYSICAL BODY
(ANNAMAYA)

THE VITAL BODY
(PRANAMAYA)

THE HEART CENTER
(ANANDAMAYA)

Cosmos
Humanity
Society
Family

THE INTELLECTUAL
MIND (MANOMAYA)

THE PERSONALITY
(VIJNANAMAYA)

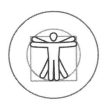

ANNAMAYA (THE PHYSICAL BODY)

All aspects of the physical body must be nourished, taking into account individual needs and limitations. According to the ancients, physical health manifests in:

- No aches and pains;
- Feeling of lightness in the body;
- Ability to withstand change;
- Sense of stability and ease.

MAIN TOOL: ASANA

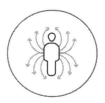

PRANAMAYA (THE VITAL BODY)

The physiological functioning is affected by the flow of prana along its five major currents: prana, apana, vyana, samana and udana. The balanced flow of prana is reflected in:

- Organ function;
- Sleep patterns;
- Stress management;
- Energy and vitality.

MAIN TOOL: PRANAYAMA, BREATH-CENTERED ASANA

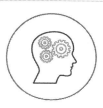

MANOMAYA (THE INTELLECTUAL MIND)

The intellectual mind has tremendous power to influence the entire system; it needs to be educated and developed to be able to:

- Direct and maintain attention;
- Make educated choices;
- Acquire knowledge (Learning);
- Retain information (Memory).

MAIN TOOLS: CHANT, TEXT STUDY

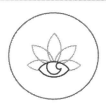

VIJNANAMAYA (THE PERSONALITY)

The personality is formed based on inherent tendencies and is affected by our experience and conditioning. It has great potential for transformation; the chakra model can be used as a road map to help us become more:

- Spiritual
- Intuitive, wise
- Expressive, truthful
- Loving, connected
- Powerful, decisive;
- Vital, creative
- Stable, secure

MAIN TOOLS: MEDITATION, SELF-REFLECTION

ANANDAMAYA (THE HEART CENTER)

The dimension of the heart is the deepest and the most profound. Through the heart we are able to relate to others and find joy and fulfillment. Ultimately, it can become a source of unconditional happiness by connecting to something greater then ourselves.

It reflects how we relate to:

- Family;
- Society;
- Humanity;
- Cosmos.

MAIN TOOLS: RITUAL, PRAYER

THE AGE MODEL

According to the viniyoga tradition, our aging process is represented by the movement of the sun throughout the day. Sunrise represents childhood, midday represents adult life, and sunset represents old age. There are specific yoga practices that are appropriate for each stage of life.

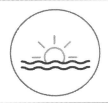 From the traditional point of view, students in a **SUNRISE STAGE** of life (teenagers and young adults) need to focus on stronger asana to help develop the growing bodies, teach discipline and encourage the body awareness.

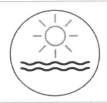 Students in a **MID-DAY STAGE** of life (roughly 25-70 years old) need more focus on the breath and other energy management practices to support them in their busy lives that likely include careers, children and households.

 Students in a **SUNSET** of life (roughly 70-80 years old and beyond) need to focus on physical maintenance and spiritual introspection to gradually turn away from the external material world and start preparing for the eventual graceful exit.

Most of us are in the "householder," or mid-day, stage of life. We are busy with responsibilities, juggling careers, children, aging parents and all the other things that come with adulthood. What we need most is stability at every level – structural stability to keep the body healthy; physiological immunity to keep us resilient; emotional balance to manage all the challenges that come our way; and financial stability to provide for ourselves and our families. This means that for the majority of us pranayama and other energy management practices are of most importance and asana is secondary.

Those of us who have moved from the "householder" to the "renunciate" stage need to focus on meditation, prayer and spiritual reflection, along with other practices appropriate for the elderly. This is a time of reflection on one's life and purpose to prepare for eventual merging back with the Source. Far from morbid, this is the time for greatest wisdom, disassociation from the material world and deep connection to something greater than one's self.

HOW TO GET THE MOST OUT OF YOUR YOGA PRACTICE
CHECKLIST

SHOW UP
First physically, literally getting down on your mat, and then mentally, bringing your attention to this moment, to this body.

LISTEN
Notice how you feel and which parts of you need more care on any given day (physical body, energy or mental state).

CONNECT TO THE BREATH
Have you breath inform and guide EVERY SINGLE ONE of your movements.

CHOOSE A PRACTICE THAT IS RELEVANT TO YOU
Short-term practices address help you deal with today's challenges.
Long-term practices address chronic issues.

KEEP YOUR ATTENTION ANCHORED
Learn how to direct and maintain attention; as it drifts away practice bringing it back.

DO MORE THAN ASANA
At a minimum, take 12 deep breaths at the end of the practice, then stay mindful of your experience for 5 minutes.

TAKE TIME TO ABSORB AND INTEGRATE
Take time between poses to close your eyes and check in with yourself. At the end, take time to observe the impact of the practice on each one of your layers.

TEN TYPES OF YOGA PRACTICES

There are many ideas out there about what a yoga practice should look like: some believe that it's only valid if it has a spiritual component, others focus on strictly physical benefits. In reality, it depends on the situation, the student and the intention. An appropriate yoga practice can facilitate change on any level – physical, physiological, spiritual - but that doesn't mean that every practice should have all those elements present. Sometimes it IS just about the body. Other times it IS all about connecting to something greater. What makes it a yoga practice is mindful movement and deep connection to the breath.

In addition, every yoga practice must be purposeful. Here are some common types of practices based on the things that we want to accomplish:

GENERAL YOGA PRACTICE
(is usually used for "flossing")

This is about moving the spine and most joints through the full range of motion, attending to most body parts without focusing on anything specific, deepening the breath and focusing the mind. The purpose here is to work toward overall balance.

FLOW PRACTICE
(links poses into "flows")

The Sun Salutation sequence is often the base of the flow practice, but it doesn't have to be. Flow practices tend to be more challenging, mostly because of the pace, and often put repetitive stress on the joints (shoulders, hips, wrists), if not sequenced mindfully.

GOAL POSTURE PRACTICE
(prepares for any complex posture)

This is about selecting a more difficult posture and then organizing the entire practice to prepare and compensate for it. The goal posture might work a specific body area, move the energy in a certain way, represent some idea, or challenge the body in a different way.

BODY PART-SPECIFIC PRACTICE
(targets neck, lower back, hips, etc.)

This addresses a specific part of the body. There can be emphasis on stretching or strengthening the area and sequencing is EXTREMELY important here if we want the practice to be effective and safe.

TEN TYPES OF YOGA PRACTICES

PRACTICE FOR A SPECIFIC ACTIVITY
(for gardening, skiing, hiking, long car drives)

This is designed either to prepare the body for an activity or compensate for the activity afterwards. These practices involve analyzing the biomechanics of the activity and need to be short and specific.

POPULATION-SPECIFIC PRACTICE
(for office workers, pregnant women, seniors)

This is designed to serve a specific group of students. We begin by analyzing the unique challenges of the students in a group and then design yoga practice(s) that meet their needs.

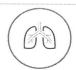

BREATH-CENTERED PRACTICE
(affects physiological functioning)

This type of practice is essential if we want to address issues with sleep, stress and energy. Here, breath adaptation and/or pranayama become central, which means that all other elements should be less complex and work to support the main element.

ENERGY-CENTERED PRACTICE
(builds or reduces energy)

This can be an energy-building practice (brhmana) or a practice that will eliminate/reduce excess energy (langhana). Working with breath is central to this type of practice, as is choosing specific yogic elements that have brhmana/langhana qualities.

INTEGRATIVE YOGA PRACTICE
(impacts the student on several layers)

Integrative practice might include chanting, meditation, visualization, ritual or prayer. Designed skillfully, they have the potential to affect the student in a more profound way, because they reach across multiple levels of the human system.

THERAPEUTIC PRACTICE
(addresses specific physical, physiological and emotional issues)

Since they are mostly created for vulnerable students with serious health challenges, teachers usually require advanced training to be able to design and teach safe and effective therapeutic practices.

ADDITIONAL RESOURCES

Would you like to know how to design each one of Ten Types of Yoga Practices?

Visit sequencewiz.org/journal to get detailed descriptions of each type of practice with handy printable infographics. Scan the code to go directly to the page. You will also find more information about the Panchamaya model and many other yoga-related topics.

SEQUENCE WIZ provides continuing education and support to yoga teachers in their personal and professional yoga journey.

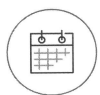 WEEKLY YOGA BLOG features articles about yoga for your body, energy and mind. The subjects of the blog range from therapeutic applications of yoga and client assessment to yoga practice sequencing, teaching tips and yoga sutras.

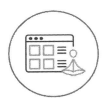 YOGA SEQUENCE BUILDER helps yoga teachers easily design yoga practices online using customizable stick figure images. It features a huge database of yoga poses, a library of predesigned practices, exclusive video series and other perks.

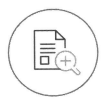 INFORMATIONAL MATERIALS include printouts of the most popular posts, infographics and leaflets about various yoga topics including yoga anatomy and physiology, yoga models, techniques and best practices.

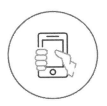 HOME YOGA PRACTICE MOBILE APP supports your home yoga practice and inspires your teaching. It addresses your physical, energetic and mental-emotional needs. The collection of videos is regularly updated to add more practices.

Today's date *August 26, 2017*   Time *7am*

How do I feel today?   *Feel kind of icky, but cannot put my finger on it*

• Physically   *Hips are tight and the lower back is a bit sore*

• Energetically   *Tired, need to perk up*

• Mentally/Emotionally   *All over the place, hard to focus*

What do I want to work on?   *Need to warm up hips and back, bring energy up,*

focus the mind and get comfortable where I am even if it is not pleasant.

What type of practice would work best today?

☐ General/Flow   ☐ Goal-posture   ☐ Body-part specific   ☐ Specific activity

☐ Breath-centered   ☐ Energy-centered   ☑ Integrative   ☐ Therapeutic

Type/Topic *Good space – bad space practice (sukha – dukha)*

What elements do I need to include?

☑ Asana   *Backbends and external hip rotation*

☑ Breath awareness/Pranayama   *Deepen Inhale, add hold after Inhale*

☑ Meditation/Reflection   *Everything that is felt needs to be*

☐ Text study   *experienced (good or bad).*

☑ Chanting   *IN(mentally): Sukha dukha*

☐ Ritual/Prayer   *EX(mentally): Good space, bad space*

☐ Other

13

MY YOGA PRACTICE: Sequence

Intention   *Become more comfortable in the body and in the current*

situation

Source   *One of my old practices from the Yoga Sutra series*

	IN(mentally): Sukha dukha *EX(mentally): Good space, bad space*
	Free breath
4 breaths	*IN(mentally): Sukha dukha* *EX(mentally): Good space, bad space*
IN EX *Stay 4br*	*Repeat 4x breathing deeply; while holding the pose, chant same as above*
IN EX *Stay 4br*	*Repeat 4x breathing deeply; while holding the pose, chant same as above*
EX IN *Stay 4br*	*Repeat 4x breathing deeply; while holding the pose, chant same as above*
EX IN *Stay 4br*	*Repeat 4x breathing deeply; while holding the pose, chant same as above*
EX IN *Stay 4br*	*Repeat 4x breathing deeply; while holding the pose, chant same as above. Then switch sides.*
IN EX *Stay 6br*	*Repeat 4x breathing deeply; while holding the pose, chant same as above. Then switch sides.*

14

IN → ← EX Stay 4br	Repeat 4x breathing deeply; then stay in the pose relaxing and breathing deeply.
	Repeat 3x breathing deeply.
Stay	Stay in the pose, chant same as above.
EX → ← IN Stay 4br	Repeat 4x breathing deeply; then stay in the pose relaxing and breathing deeply.
Stay 4 br	Stay in the pose, chant same as above; then move to the next pose on the same side.
Stay 6br	Stay in the pose, chant same as above. Then do both poses on the other side.
IN → ← EX Stay 6br	Repeat 4x breathing deeply; then stay in the pose relaxing and breathing deeply.
	Rest.
12 br	Pranayama. IN(mentally): Sukha – good space; HOLD EX(mentally): Dukha – bad space /12 br
10 min	Meditation: sensory awareness. Notice the sounds, smells, tactile sensations, position in space. Stay present with it.

15

Notes and reflections

At first there was a lot of physical and mental resistance, breathing felt restricted. Little by little it eased off. It helped to chant mentally while holding the pose to both keep the breath a steady pace and overcome physical resistance in the pose. The practice felt like it was a good length and pretty balanced; it did help loosen up the hips and back. It worked well to change the chant in Pranayama both to keep the IN a bit longer and to hold my attention. Sensory awareness meditation was really effective in anchoring me in the present moment (especially focusing on the sounds). It helped me realize that this moment is neither good nor bad; it is my perception that makes it so. For a few minutes I was able to let go of my mental coloring and just stay fully aware of my sensory input.

It felt clarifying for the mind.

Overall the practice was effective, but may be next time I will experiment with a different Pranayama to impact the energy a bit more. May be Krama Inhale? Or may be I just need a good night' s sleep ☺

The practice took about 50 minutes.

PERSONAL YOGA PRACTICE
JOURNAL

....

....

....

30 DAYS OF YOGA PLANNER

30 DAYS OF YOGA PLANNER

Notes

Today's date _____   Time _____

How do I feel today? _____

• Physically _____

• Energetically _____

• Mentally/Emotionally _____

What do I want to work on? _____

What type of practice would work best today?

☐ General/Flow   ☐ Goal-posture   ☐ Body-part specific   ☐ Specific activity

☐ Breath-centered   ☐ Energy-centered   ☐ Integrative   ☐ Therapeutic

Type/Topic

What elements do I need to include?

☐ Asana

☐ Breath awareness/Pranayama

☐ Meditation/Reflection

☐ Text study

☐ Chanting

☐ Ritual/Prayer

☐ Other

21

Intention

Source

Notes and reflections

Today's date _____   Time _____

MY YOGA PRACTICE: Before practice

How do I feel today?

- Physically _____

- Energetically _____

- Mentally/Emotionally _____

What do I want to work on? _____

What type of practice would work best today?

☐ General/Flow   ☐ Goal-posture   ☐ Body-part specific   ☐ Specific activity

☐ Breath-centered   ☐ Energy-centered   ☐ Integrative   ☐ Therapeutic

Type/Topic

What elements do I need to include?

☐ Asana

☐ Breath awareness/Pranayama

☐ Meditation/Reflection

☐ Text study

☐ Chanting

☐ Ritual/Prayer

☐ Other

Intention

Source

Notes and reflections

Today's date _____   Time _____

How do I feel today?

- Physically _____

- Energetically _____

- Mentally/Emotionally _____

What do I want to work on? _____

_____

What type of practice would work best today?

☐ General/Flow   ☐ Goal-posture   ☐ Body-part specific   ☐ Specific activity

☐ Breath-centered   ☐ Energy-centered   ☐ Integrative   ☐ Therapeutic

Type/Topic

What elements do I need to include?

☐ Asana

☐ Breath awareness/Pranayama

☐ Meditation/Reflection

☐ Text study

☐ Chanting

☐ Ritual/Prayer

☐ Other

Intention

Source

Notes and reflections

Today's date _____ Time _____

How do I feel today?

• Physically _____

• Energetically _____

• Mentally/Emotionally _____

What do I want to work on? _____

What type of practice would work best today?

☐ General/Flow   ☐ Goal-posture   ☐ Body-part specific   ☐ Specific activity

☐ Breath-centered   ☐ Energy-centered   ☐ Integrative   ☐ Therapeutic

Type/Topic

What elements do I need to include?

☐ Asana

☐ Breath awareness/Pranayama

☐ Meditation/Reflection

☐ Text study

☐ Chanting

☐ Ritual/Prayer

☐ Other

Intention

Source

Notes and reflections

Today's date _____   Time _____

How do I feel today?

• Physically _____

• Energetically _____

• Mentally/Emotionally _____

What do I want to work on? _____

What type of practice would work best today?

☐ General/Flow   ☐ Goal-posture   ☐ Body-part specific   ☐ Specific activity

☐ Breath-centered   ☐ Energy-centered   ☐ Integrative   ☐ Therapeutic

Type/Topic

What elements do I need to include?

☐ Asana

☐ Breath awareness/Pranayama

☐ Meditation/Reflection

☐ Text study

☐ Chanting

☐ Ritual/Prayer

☐ Other

Intention

Source

Notes and reflections

Today's date _____   Time _____

MY YOGA PRACTICE: Before practice

How do I feel today?   _____

• Physically   _____

• Energetically   _____

• Mentally/Emotionally   _____

What do I want to work on?   _____

_____

What type of practice would work best today?

☐ General/Flow   ☐ Goal-posture   ☐ Body-part specific   ☐ Specific activity

☐ Breath-centered   ☐ Energy-centered   ☐ Integrative   ☐ Therapeutic

Type/Topic

What elements do I need to include?

☐ Asana

☐ Breath awareness/Pranayama

☐ Meditation/Reflection

☐ Text study

☐ Chanting

☐ Ritual/Prayer

☐ Other

Intention

Source

Notes and reflections

Today's date _____   Time _____

How do I feel today? _____

• Physically _____

• Energetically _____

• Mentally/Emotionally _____

What do I want to work on? _____

_____

What type of practice would work best today?

☐ General/Flow   ☐ Goal-posture   ☐ Body-part specific   ☐ Specific activity

☐ Breath-centered   ☐ Energy-centered   ☐ Integrative   ☐ Therapeutic

Type/Topic

What elements do I need to include?

☐ Asana

☐ Breath awareness/Pranayama

☐ Meditation/Reflection

☐ Text study

☐ Chanting

☐ Ritual/Prayer

☐ Other

Intention

Source

Notes and reflections

Today's date _____   Time _____

How do I feel today?

- Physically _____

- Energetically _____

- Mentally/Emotionally _____

What do I want to work on? _____

What type of practice would work best today?

☐ General/Flow   ☐ Goal-posture   ☐ Body-part specific   ☐ Specific activity

☐ Breath-centered   ☐ Energy-centered   ☐ Integrative   ☐ Therapeutic

Type/Topic

What elements do I need to include?

☐ Asana

☐ Breath awareness/Pranayama

☐ Meditation/Reflection

☐ Text study

☐ Chanting

☐ Ritual/Prayer

☐ Other

Intention

Source

Notes and reflections

Today's date _____   Time _____

How do I feel today?

• Physically _____

• Energetically _____

• Mentally/Emotionally _____

What do I want to work on? _____

_____

What type of practice would work best today?

☐ General/Flow ☐ Goal-posture ☐ Body-part specific ☐ Specific activity

☐ Breath-centered ☐ Energy-centered ☐ Integrative ☐ Therapeutic

Type/Topic _____

What elements do I need to include?

☐ Asana

☐ Breath awareness/Pranayama

☐ Meditation/Reflection

☐ Text study

☐ Chanting

☐ Ritual/Prayer

☐ Other

Intention

Source

Notes and reflections

Today's date _____   Time _____

How do I feel today?

• Physically

• Energetically

• Mentally/Emotionally

What do I want to work on?

What type of practice would work best today?

☐ General/Flow ☐ Goal-posture ☐ Body-part specific ☐ Specific activity

☐ Breath-centered ☐ Energy-centered ☐ Integrative ☐ Therapeutic

Type/Topic

What elements do I need to include?

☐ Asana

☐ Breath awareness/Pranayama

☐ Meditation/Reflection

☐ Text study

☐ Chanting

☐ Ritual/Prayer

☐ Other

Intention

Source

Notes and reflections

Today's date _____   Time _____

How do I feel today? _____

• Physically _____

• Energetically _____

• Mentally/Emotionally _____

What do I want to work on? _____

_____

What type of practice would work best today?

☐ General/Flow   ☐ Goal-posture   ☐ Body-part specific   ☐ Specific activity

☐ Breath-centered   ☐ Energy-centered   ☐ Integrative   ☐ Therapeutic

Type/Topic

What elements do I need to include?

☐ Asana

☐ Breath awareness/Pranayama

☐ Meditation/Reflection

☐ Text study

☐ Chanting

☐ Ritual/Prayer

☐ Other

Intention

Source

Notes and reflections

Today's date _____   Time _____

MY YOGA PRACTICE: Before practice

How do I feel today?   ....

• Physically   ....

• Energetically   ....

• Mentally/Emotionally   ....

What do I want to work on?   ....

What type of practice would work best today?

☐ General/Flow   ☐ Goal-posture   ☐ Body-part specific   ☐ Specific activity

☐ Breath-centered   ☐ Energy-centered   ☐ Integrative   ☐ Therapeutic

Type/Topic

What elements do I need to include?

☐ Asana   ....

☐ Breath awareness/Pranayama

☐ Meditation/Reflection

☐ Text study

☐ Chanting

☐ Ritual/Prayer

☐ Other

Intention

Source

Notes and reflections

Today's date _____   Time _____

How do I feel today?

• Physically

• Energetically

• Mentally/Emotionally

What do I want to work on?

What type of practice would work best today?

☐ General/Flow   ☐ Goal-posture   ☐ Body-part specific   ☐ Specific activity

☐ Breath-centered   ☐ Energy-centered   ☐ Integrative   ☐ Therapeutic

Type/Topic

What elements do I need to include?

☐ Asana

☐ Breath awareness/Pranayama

☐ Meditation/Reflection

☐ Text study

☐ Chanting

☐ Ritual/Prayer

☐ Other

Intention

Source

Notes and reflections

Today's date _____   Time _____

How do I feel today?

- Physically _____

- Energetically _____

- Mentally/Emotionally _____

What do I want to work on? _____

What type of practice would work best today?

☐ General/Flow   ☐ Goal-posture   ☐ Body-part specific   ☐ Specific activity

☐ Breath-centered   ☐ Energy-centered   ☐ Integrative   ☐ Therapeutic

Type/Topic

What elements do I need to include?

☐ Asana

☐ Breath awareness/Pranayama

☐ Meditation/Reflection

☐ Text study

☐ Chanting

☐ Ritual/Prayer

☐ Other

Intention

Source

Notes and reflections

Today's date _____   Time _____

How do I feel today?

- Physically

- Energetically

- Mentally/Emotionally

What do I want to work on?

What type of practice would work best today?

☐ General/Flow   ☐ Goal-posture   ☐ Body-part specific   ☐ Specific activity

☐ Breath-centered   ☐ Energy-centered   ☐ Integrative   ☐ Therapeutic

Type/Topic

What elements do I need to include?

☐ Asana

☐ Breath awareness/Pranayama

☐ Meditation/Reflection

☐ Text study

☐ Chanting

☐ Ritual/Prayer

☐ Other

Intention

Source

Notes and reflections

Today's date _____   Time _____

How do I feel today? _____

• Physically _____

• Energetically _____

• Mentally/Emotionally _____

What do I want to work on? _____

_____

What type of practice would work best today?

☐ General/Flow   ☐ Goal-posture   ☐ Body-part specific   ☐ Specific activity

☐ Breath-centered   ☐ Energy-centered   ☐ Integrative   ☐ Therapeutic

Type/Topic _____

_____

What elements do I need to include?

☐ Asana

☐ Breath awareness/Pranayama

☐ Meditation/Reflection

☐ Text study

☐ Chanting

☐ Ritual/Prayer

☐ Other

Intention

Source

Notes and reflections

Today's date _____   Time _____

How do I feel today? _____

• Physically _____

• Energetically _____

• Mentally/Emotionally _____

What do I want to work on? _____

What type of practice would work best today?

☐ General/Flow   ☐ Goal-posture   ☐ Body-part specific   ☐ Specific activity

☐ Breath-centered   ☐ Energy-centered   ☐ Integrative   ☐ Therapeutic

Type/Topic _____

What elements do I need to include?

☐ Asana

☐ Breath awareness/Pranayama

☐ Meditation/Reflection

☐ Text study

☐ Chanting

☐ Ritual/Prayer

☐ Other

Intention

Source

Notes and reflections

Today's date _____ Time _____

MY YOGA PRACTICE: Before practice

How do I feel today? _____

• Physically _____

• Energetically _____

• Mentally/Emotionally _____

What do I want to work on? _____

What type of practice would work best today?

☐ General/Flow   ☐ Goal-posture   ☐ Body-part specific   ☐ Specific activity

☐ Breath-centered   ☐ Energy-centered   ☐ Integrative   ☐ Therapeutic

Type/Topic _____

What elements do I need to include?

☐ Asana

☐ Breath awareness/Pranayama

☐ Meditation/Reflection

☐ Text study

☐ Chanting

☐ Ritual/Prayer

☐ Other

Intention

Source

Notes and reflections

Today's date _____   Time _____

How do I feel today?

• Physically

• Energetically

• Mentally/Emotionally

What do I want to work on?

What type of practice would work best today?

☐ General/Flow   ☐ Goal-posture   ☐ Body-part specific   ☐ Specific activity

☐ Breath-centered   ☐ Energy-centered   ☐ Integrative   ☐ Therapeutic

Type/Topic

What elements do I need to include?

☐ Asana

☐ Breath awareness/Pranayama

☐ Meditation/Reflection

☐ Text study

☐ Chanting

☐ Ritual/Prayer

☐ Other

Intention

Source

Notes and reflections

Today's date _____   Time _____

How do I feel today? _____

• Physically _____

• Energetically _____

• Mentally/Emotionally _____

What do I want to work on? _____

_____

What type of practice would work best today?

☐ General/Flow ☐ Goal-posture ☐ Body-part specific ☐ Specific activity

☐ Breath-centered ☐ Energy-centered ☐ Integrative ☐ Therapeutic

Type/Topic

What elements do I need to include?

☐ Asana

☐ Breath awareness/Pranayama

☐ Meditation/Reflection

☐ Text study

☐ Chanting

☐ Ritual/Prayer

☐ Other

Intention

Source

Notes and reflections

Today's date _____   Time _____

How do I feel today?

- Physically _____

- Energetically _____

- Mentally/Emotionally _____

What do I want to work on? _____

What type of practice would work best today?

☐ General/Flow ☐ Goal-posture ☐ Body-part specific ☐ Specific activity

☐ Breath-centered ☐ Energy-centered ☐ Integrative ☐ Therapeutic

Type/Topic

What elements do I need to include?

☐ Asana

☐ Breath awareness/Pranayama

☐ Meditation/Reflection

☐ Text study

☐ Chanting

☐ Ritual/Prayer

☐ Other

Intention

Source

Notes and reflections

Today's date _____   Time _____

How do I feel today? _____

• Physically _____

• Energetically _____

• Mentally/Emotionally _____

What do I want to work on? _____

_____

What type of practice would work best today?

☐ General/Flow   ☐ Goal-posture   ☐ Body-part specific   ☐ Specific activity

☐ Breath-centered   ☐ Energy-centered   ☐ Integrative   ☐ Therapeutic

Type/Topic

What elements do I need to include?

☐ Asana

☐ Breath awareness/Pranayama

☐ Meditation/Reflection

☐ Text study

☐ Chanting

☐ Ritual/Prayer

☐ Other

Intention

Source

Notes and reflections

Today's date _____   Time _____

MY YOGA PRACTICE: Before practice

How do I feel today? _____

• Physically _____

• Energetically _____

• Mentally/Emotionally _____

What do I want to work on? _____

What type of practice would work best today?

☐ General/Flow   ☐ Goal-posture   ☐ Body-part specific   ☐ Specific activity

☐ Breath-centered   ☐ Energy-centered   ☐ Integrative   ☐ Therapeutic

Type/Topic

What elements do I need to include?

☐ Asana

☐ Breath awareness/Pranayama

☐ Meditation/Reflection

☐ Text study

☐ Chanting

☐ Ritual/Prayer

☐ Other

Intention

Source

Notes and reflections

Today's date _____   Time _____

How do I feel today? _____

• Physically _____

• Energetically _____

• Mentally/Emotionally _____

What do I want to work on? _____

_____

_____

What type of practice would work best today?

☐ General/Flow   ☐ Goal-posture   ☐ Body-part specific   ☐ Specific activity

☐ Breath-centered   ☐ Energy-centered   ☐ Integrative   ☐ Therapeutic

Type/Topic _____

_____

What elements do I need to include?

☐ Asana

☐ Breath awareness/Pranayama

☐ Meditation/Reflection

☐ Text study

☐ Chanting

☐ Ritual/Prayer

☐ Other

Intention

Source

Notes and reflections

Today's date _____ Time _____

How do I feel today? _____

• Physically _____

• Energetically _____

• Mentally/Emotionally _____

What do I want to work on? _____

_____

What type of practice would work best today?

☐ General/Flow   ☐ Goal-posture   ☐ Body-part specific   ☐ Specific activity

☐ Breath-centered   ☐ Energy-centered   ☐ Integrative   ☐ Therapeutic

Type/Topic

What elements do I need to include?

☐ Asana

☐ Breath awareness/Pranayama

☐ Meditation/Reflection

☐ Text study

☐ Chanting

☐ Ritual/Prayer

☐ Other

Intention

Source

Notes and reflections

Today's date _____   Time _____

How do I feel today?

• Physically _____

• Energetically _____

• Mentally/Emotionally _____

What do I want to work on? _____

What type of practice would work best today?

☐ General/Flow ☐ Goal-posture ☐ Body-part specific ☐ Specific activity

☐ Breath-centered ☐ Energy-centered ☐ Integrative ☐ Therapeutic

Type/Topic

What elements do I need to include?

☐ Asana

☐ Breath awareness/Pranayama

☐ Meditation/Reflection

☐ Text study

☐ Chanting

☐ Ritual/Prayer

☐ Other

Intention

Source

Notes and reflections

Today's date _____   Time _____

MY YOGA PRACTICE: Before practice

How do I feel today?

• Physically

• Energetically

• Mentally/Emotionally

What do I want to work on?

What type of practice would work best today?

☐ General/Flow   ☐ Goal-posture   ☐ Body-part specific   ☐ Specific activity

☐ Breath-centered   ☐ Energy-centered   ☐ Integrative   ☐ Therapeutic

Type/Topic

What elements do I need to include?

☐ Asana

☐ Breath awareness/Pranayama

☐ Meditation/Reflection

☐ Text study

☐ Chanting

☐ Ritual/Prayer

☐ Other

Intention

Source

Notes and reflections

Today's date _____   Time _____

How do I feel today?   _____

• Physically   _____

• Energetically   _____

• Mentally/Emotionally   _____

What do I want to work on?   _____

What type of practice would work best today?

☐ General/Flow   ☐ Goal-posture   ☐ Body-part specific   ☐ Specific activity

☐ Breath-centered   ☐ Energy-centered   ☐ Integrative   ☐ Therapeutic

Type/Topic

What elements do I need to include?

☐ Asana

☐ Breath awareness/Pranayama

☐ Meditation/Reflection

☐ Text study

☐ Chanting

☐ Ritual/Prayer

☐ Other

Intention

Source

Notes and reflections

Today's date _____   Time _____

MY YOGA PRACTICE: Before practice

How do I feel today?   _____

• Physically   _____

• Energetically   _____

• Mentally/Emotionally   _____

What do I want to work on?   _____

What type of practice would work best today?

☐ General/Flow   ☐ Goal-posture   ☐ Body-part specific   ☐ Specific activity

☐ Breath-centered   ☐ Energy-centered   ☐ Integrative   ☐ Therapeutic

Type/Topic

What elements do I need to include?

☐ Asana

☐ Breath awareness/Pranayama

☐ Meditation/Reflection

☐ Text study

☐ Chanting

☐ Ritual/Prayer

☐ Other

Intention

Source

Notes and reflections

Today's date _____   Time _____

How do I feel today? _____

• Physically _____

• Energetically _____

• Mentally/Emotionally _____

What do I want to work on? _____

What type of practice would work best today?

☐ General/Flow   ☐ Goal-posture   ☐ Body-part specific   ☐ Specific activity

☐ Breath-centered   ☐ Energy-centered   ☐ Integrative   ☐ Therapeutic

Type/Topic

What elements do I need to include?

☐ Asana

☐ Breath awareness/Pranayama

☐ Meditation/Reflection

☐ Text study

☐ Chanting

☐ Ritual/Prayer

☐ Other

Intention

Source

Notes and reflections

Made in the USA
Lexington, KY
20 September 2017